Lose Weight, Gain Health:

Your Journey to a Better You

DR. MELISSA P. NELSON

TABLE OF CONTENTS

INTRODUCTION

Welcome to "Lose Weight, Gain Health: Your Journey to a Better You." This book is a comprehensive guide designed to empower and support you on your transformative path towards a healthier and happier life. Whether you're seeking to shed extra pounds, boost your energy levels, or improve your overall well-being, this journey is about much more than just losing weight; it's about gaining a deeper understanding of yourself and nurturing a positive relationship with your body.

In a world where quick fixes and fad diets abound, it's easy to feel overwhelmed and lost on your quest for a sustainable and effective weight loss strategy. But fear not, for this book is here to be your steadfast companion throughout your transformation. Together, we will explore the power of mindful eating, the benefits of regular physical activity, and the importance of nurturing your mental and emotional well-being. Along the way, you'll discover practical tips, actionable steps, and evidence-based strategies to make lasting changes in your life.

Your journey to a better you is a personal and unique one. It's about embracing progress over perfection and celebrating every milestone, no matter how small. Throughout this book, we will delve into the art of self-compassion, understanding that setbacks are a natural part of the process, and that each step forward is a victory worth celebrating.

This book is not about strict rules or deprivation; it's about empowerment and choice. You hold the reins to your journey, and we will equip you with the tools to make informed decisions that align with your goals and values. As you embark on this path of transformation, remember that it's not just about reaching a destination but embracing the beauty of the journey itself.

So, let's begin this incredible expedition to discover the best version of yourself. Together, we will embrace the joy of mindful eating, find fulfillment in physical activity, and cultivate a positive relationship with your body and mind. Let this book be your guiding light, your source of inspiration, and your unwavering companion as you embark on the remarkable journey to lose weight, gain health, and become the best version of you. The adventure awaits!

CHAPTER 1: UNDERSTANDING WEIGHT LOSS AND HEALTH

In today's fast-paced world, maintaining a healthy weight has become increasingly important for overall well-being. Our weight not only impacts our physical appearance but also plays a vital role in determining our overall health and quality of life. This chapter will delve into the significance of a healthy weight and its profound effects on our well-being.

The Importance Of A Healthy Weight For Overall Well-being

Maintaining a healthy weight is crucial for overall well-being as it significantly impacts various aspects of our physical and mental health. Firstly, it reduces the risk of chronic health conditions, such as heart disease, type 2 diabetes, hypertension, and certain cancers. Excess weight puts strain on the heart and other organs, leading to an increased likelihood of developing these conditions.

Secondly, a healthy weight promotes better joint health and mobility, as excessive weight can lead to joint pain and increased wear and tear on the joints. By maintaining a healthy weight, individuals can improve their ability to move comfortably and engage in physical activities.

Moreover, achieving and maintaining a healthy weight contributes to improved energy levels and overall vitality. Excess body fat can lead to fatigue and decreased stamina, affecting daily activities and reducing quality of life. On the other hand, a healthy weight fosters a sense of well-being, enhances self-esteem, and boosts confidence.

Furthermore, weight plays a role in mental health. Negative body image and low self-esteem resulting from being overweight or underweight can lead to psychological distress. Striving for a healthy weight, coupled with positive body image, promotes better mental well-being and may reduce the risk of developing eating disorders.

Overall, a healthy weight is essential for maximizing one's overall well-being, preventing chronic illnesses, promoting physical activity, enhancing self-esteem, and supporting mental health. It is crucial to adopt a balanced approach to weight management, incorporating a nutritious diet, regular exercise, and sustainable lifestyle changes for long-term health benefits.

The Relationship Between Weight Loss And Improved Health

The relationship between weight loss and improved health is well-established and supported by extensive research. Shedding excess weight can lead to a range of health benefits that positively impact various aspects of our well-being.

Reduced Risk of Chronic Diseases: Weight loss has been linked to a decreased risk of chronic health conditions such as cardiovascular disease, type 2 diabetes, and certain types of cancer. By managing weight, individuals can lower their blood pressure, improve cholesterol levels, and reduce inflammation, all of which contribute to a healthier cardiovascular system.

Better Glucose Regulation: Losing weight can enhance insulin sensitivity and glucose regulation, which is crucial for preventing and managing type 2 diabetes. Weight loss, especially through healthy lifestyle changes, can help control blood sugar levels and decrease the need for diabetes medication.

Improved Joint Health: Excess weight puts extra stress on the joints, leading to joint pain and an increased risk of conditions like osteoarthritis. Weight loss reduces the burden on the joints, leading to improved mobility and reduced discomfort.

Enhanced Respiratory Function: Weight loss can improve lung function and reduce the risk of respiratory problems. Obesity is associated with conditions like sleep apnea, which can be alleviated or even resolved through weight loss.

Mental Well-being: Weight loss can have positive effects on mental health, including increased self-esteem and reduced symptoms of depression and anxiety. Feeling more confident in one's body and achieving personal health goals can boost overall mood and emotional well-being.

Increased Energy Levels: Shedding excess weight can lead to increased energy levels and greater stamina for physical activities. This, in turn, encourages individuals to be more active, creating a positive feedback loop that further supports weight management and overall health.

Lowered Inflammation: Obesity is associated with chronic inflammation, which is linked to various health issues. Weight loss has been shown to reduce markers of inflammation, potentially decreasing the risk of inflammatory-related diseases.

It is important to note that weight loss should be approached in a healthy and sustainable manner, avoiding crash diets or extreme measures. A balanced combination of a nutritious diet, regular exercise, and lifestyle changes tailored to individual needs and preferences is key to achieving and maintaining weight loss while promoting improved overall health. Consulting with healthcare professionals or registered dietitians can provide personalized guidance and support on the weight loss journey.

Debunking Common Myths And Misconceptions About Weight Loss

Debunking common myths and misconceptions about weight loss is essential to help individuals make informed decisions and adopt a realistic and effective approach to managing their weight.
Let's explore some of these myths:

1. Myth: Quick-fix diets lead to long-term weight loss.

Fact: Quick-fix diets, often promising rapid results, are usually unsustainable and can be harmful to overall health. Successful weight loss requires gradual, sustainable lifestyle changes like a balanced diet and regular exercise.

2. Myth: Skipping meals helps in losing weight.

Fact: Skipping meals can disrupt metabolism, lead to nutrient deficiencies, and encourage overeating later in the day. Eating regular, well-portioned meals is key to a balanced and healthy approach to weight management.

3. Myth: Carbohydrates are always bad for weight loss.

Fact: Carbohydrates are an essential source of energy and can be part of a healthy weight loss plan. Choosing complex carbs like whole grains, fruits, and vegetables is beneficial for sustained energy levels and overall health.

4. Myth: You must avoid all fats to lose weight.

Fact: Not all fats are bad. Healthy fats, such as those found in avocados, nuts, and olive oil, are crucial for various bodily functions and can even support weight loss when consumed in moderation.

5. Myth: You can spot-reduce fat in specific areas.

Fact: Spot reduction is a myth. Fat loss occurs throughout the body, and targeted exercises may tone specific muscles but won't lead to fat loss in those areas alone.

6. Myth: Weight loss supplements are a magic solution.

Fact: Weight loss supplements are often not backed by substantial evidence and may come with potential side effects. Sustainable weight loss is best achieved through a balanced diet and regular exercise.

7. Myth: All calories are equal.

Fact: While calorie intake matters for weight loss, the quality of those calories is also crucial. Nutrient-dense foods that provide essential vitamins and minerals are better for overall health and satiety.

8. Myth: Crash diets are a safe way to lose weight quickly.

Fact: Crash diets can lead to nutritional deficiencies, muscle loss, and a slowed metabolism. They are unsustainable and can negatively impact overall health.

9. Myth: Exercise is the only factor that matters for weight loss.

Fact: Exercise is essential for overall health and can aid weight loss, but diet plays a more significant role in weight management. A combination of both is most effective.

10. Myth: Losing weight is a linear process.

Fact: Weight loss progress may vary over time due to factors like water retention, muscle gain, and hormonal fluctuations. Plateaus are common, and patience is key in a successful weight loss journey.

By debunking these myths and understanding the realities of weight loss, individuals can approach their weight management goals with a more informed and realistic perspective, leading to better long-term results and improved overall health. Consulting with healthcare professionals or registered dietitians can provide further guidance and support in developing a personalized and effective weight loss plan.

CHAPTER 2: ASSESSING YOUR CURRENT HEALTH AND HABITS

Before embarking on any weight loss journey, it is essential to assess your current health status, dietary habits, and lifestyle choices. This chapter will guide you through a comprehensive evaluation to identify your health goals, areas for improvement, and set realistic expectations for your weight loss journey.

Evaluating Your Current Weight, Diet, And Lifestyle

Assessing your current weight, diet, and lifestyle is the foundational step in any journey towards improved health and weight management. This evaluation provides valuable insights into your current state of well-being and helps identify areas that may need adjustment to achieve your health goals. Let's explore the importance of evaluating each of these aspects in detail:

Current Weight:
Knowing your current weight and body composition is essential for understanding your starting point and setting

realistic weight loss goals. Several methods can help you measure your weight, including standard bathroom scales, smart scales that provide additional body composition metrics, or body fat calipers. Keep in mind that weight alone may not fully represent your overall health, as it doesn't differentiate between fat, muscle, and water weight. Therefore, considering other measures like waist circumference and body fat percentage can offer a more comprehensive view.

Diet:

Evaluating your diet involves taking a closer look at your eating habits and nutritional intake. Keeping a food journal for a few days can be immensely helpful in this process. Record everything you eat and drink, including portion sizes and snacking habits. Analyze the types of foods you consume regularly. Are you getting enough fruits, vegetables, and whole grains? Are you consuming excessive amounts of processed or sugary foods? Identifying areas of concern will allow you to make informed choices and create a balanced and nutritious meal plan.

Lifestyle:

Your lifestyle plays a significant role in your overall health and weight management. Consider your daily routines and activity levels. Are you predominantly sedentary, or do you engage in regular physical activity? Evaluate the amount of time you spend sitting, walking, exercising, or participating in recreational activities. Additionally, examine your sleep patterns and stress levels, as they can influence your eating habits and overall health. Understanding your lifestyle habits will help you tailor a plan that fits your unique needs and preferences.

The Benefits Of Evaluation

Personalized Approach: Assessing your current weight, diet, and lifestyle allows you to design a personalized and effective health plan. Identifying areas that need improvement empowers you to make targeted changes that will have a positive impact on your well-being.

Goal Setting: Knowing where you stand allows you to set realistic and achievable health goals. Whether it's weight loss, muscle gain, or overall wellness, setting specific objectives based on your current state increases the likelihood of success.

Tracking Progress: Evaluation provides a baseline to track your progress over time. Regularly monitoring changes in your weight, dietary habits, and lifestyle helps you stay motivated and adjust your plan as needed.

Health Awareness: By evaluating your health, you become more aware of your body and its needs. This heightened awareness encourages mindful decision-making and fosters a greater sense of responsibility for your well-being.

Remember that the evaluation process is not meant to be judgmental or critical. Instead, view it as a valuable learning experience that sets the groundwork for positive changes. Seek support from healthcare professionals or certified nutritionists if needed, as they can provide expert guidance and support throughout your journey to a healthier and happier lifestyle.

Identifying Health Goals And Areas For Improvement

Setting clear and realistic health goals is a crucial step towards achieving a healthier and more fulfilling life. By identifying specific health objectives and recognizing areas that need improvement, you can develop a focused and actionable plan to enhance your well-being. Here's how to effectively identify health goals and areas for improvement:

Be Specific and Realistic:

When setting health goals, be specific about what you want to achieve. Whether it's losing a certain amount of weight, running a 5K race, or reducing stress levels, clearly define your objectives. Avoid setting overly ambitious goals that may feel unattainable, as this can lead to frustration and demotivation. Instead, choose targets that are challenging yet achievable within a reasonable timeframe.

Prioritize Your Goals:

Consider your overall well-being and determine which areas of your health need the most attention. Are you looking to improve your physical fitness, enhance your mental well-being, or manage a specific health condition? Prioritize your goals based on their importance and relevance to your current life situation.

Make Your Goals Measurable:

To track progress effectively, make your health goals measurable. Use quantifiable parameters like weight, body fat percentage, blood pressure, or exercise duration to gauge your achievements. Being able to measure your progress will help you stay on track and motivated as you witness positive changes over time.

Set Short-term and Long-term Goals:

Break down your health goals into short-term and long-term objectives. Short-term goals allow you to celebrate smaller victories along the way, while long-term goals keep you focused on the bigger picture. This approach helps maintain momentum and provides a sense of accomplishment as you work towards your ultimate aspirations.

Focus on Areas for Improvement:

Identify areas of your life that require improvement to support your health goals. This could include dietary habits, physical activity levels, stress management, sleep patterns, or even relationships. Take an honest and non-judgmental look at these areas and create strategies to address them positively.

Seek Professional Guidance:

If you're uncertain about the best approach to improve certain aspects of your health, consider seeking guidance from healthcare professionals, registered dietitians, or certified fitness trainers. They can provide expert advice, personalized recommendations, and support tailored to your unique needs.

Be Adaptable:

Life is dynamic, and circumstances may change along your health journey. Be adaptable and open to modifying your goals and strategies as needed. Flexibility allows you to navigate challenges and setbacks while staying committed to your overall health and well-being.

Remember that identifying health goals and areas for improvement is a continuous process. As you make progress and achieve your objectives, new goals may emerge, and your priorities may shift. Embrace this journey as an opportunity for growth, learning, and self-discovery, and celebrate every step towards a healthier and happier you.

Tracking Progress And Setting Realistic Expectations

Tracking progress and setting realistic expectations are integral components of any successful health and wellness journey. By monitoring your advancements and maintaining practical outlooks, you can stay motivated, focused, and empowered to achieve your health goals. Here's how to effectively track progress and establish achievable expectations:

Keep Track of Your Progress:

Regularly monitor and record your achievements, whether they relate to weight loss, fitness levels, dietary changes, or stress management. Use tools such as fitness trackers, food journals, or health apps to track relevant metrics. This allows you to objectively assess your progress over time and identify areas that may require additional attention.

Celebrate Small Victories:
Acknowledge and celebrate every small victory along the way. Whether it's consistently following a new exercise routine, making healthier food choices, or managing stress more effectively, each accomplishment deserves recognition. Celebrating these milestones boosts motivation and reinforces positive behavior changes.

Set Measurable Milestones:
Break down your long-term health goals into smaller, measurable milestones. These intermediate targets act as stepping stones towards your larger objectives. Measurable milestones provide a sense of direction and accomplishment, making the journey feel more manageable and attainable.

Be Patient and Realistic:
Patience is key when pursuing sustainable improvements in health. Understand that meaningful changes take time and

consistency. Avoid comparing your progress to others, as everyone's journey is unique. Set realistic expectations based on your individual circumstances, starting point, and desired outcomes.

Embrace Non-Scale Victories:
While tracking progress through numbers is essential, don't overlook non-scale victories. Improved energy levels, better sleep, enhanced mood, increased strength, and improved endurance are all signs of positive change, even if the scale may not reflect it immediately. Embrace these non-scale victories as important markers of progress.

Accept Setbacks and Learn from Them:
Expect that setbacks and challenges will occur during your health journey. Instead of feeling discouraged, view them as learning opportunities. Analyze the factors that led to setbacks, and use that knowledge to refine your approach and create strategies for future success.

Adjust Goals When Necessary:
As circumstances change and you gain more insight into your health and lifestyle, be willing to adjust your goals. Flexibility is essential in maintaining a sustainable and adaptive approach. Setbacks or shifts in priorities may

require modifications to your expectations, but remember that adapting your goals does not equate to failure.

Seek Support and Accountability:
Consider involving a friend, family member, or health professional as an accountability partner. Sharing your progress and challenges with someone can provide valuable support, encouragement, and motivation.

In conclusion, tracking progress and setting realistic expectations are vital aspects of your health journey. Embrace the process with patience, self-compassion, and a growth mindset. By celebrating victories, learning from setbacks, and adapting your goals when necessary, you'll create a positive and transformative path towards improved health and overall well-being.

CHAPTER 3: NUTRITION ESSENTIALS FOR WEIGHT LOSS

Nutrition is a fundamental pillar of any successful weight loss journey. In this chapter, we will delve into the essential components of nutrition for effective weight management. By creating a balanced and sustainable meal plan, understanding the role of macronutrients and micronutrients, and making healthy food choices with proper portion control, you can optimize your nutrition for weight loss and overall well-being.

Creating A Balanced And Sustainable Meal Plan

Designing a balanced and sustainable meal plan is a crucial aspect of achieving successful weight loss and maintaining overall health. A well-crafted meal plan ensures that you get all the necessary nutrients while promoting steady and sustainable progress towards your goals. Here are some key steps to create a balanced and sustainable meal plan:

Assess Your Nutritional Needs:

Start by assessing your individual nutritional needs based on factors like age, gender, weight, activity level, and health conditions. Consulting a registered dietitian or nutrition expert can provide personalized guidance to meet your specific requirements.

Include a Variety of Food Groups:
A balanced meal plan should include a variety of food groups, ensuring you receive a wide range of nutrients. Focus on incorporating the following food groups into your meals:

- **Fruits and Vegetables**: Aim for a colorful assortment of fruits and vegetables, which are rich in vitamins, minerals, and fiber.

- **Whole Grains**: Opt for whole grains like brown rice, quinoa, whole wheat, and oats, which offer more nutrients and fiber than refined grains.

- **Lean Proteins**: Include lean sources of protein such as poultry, fish, tofu, legumes, and low-fat dairy. Protein helps maintain muscle mass and keeps you feeling full.

- **Healthy Fats**: Incorporate sources of healthy fats like avocados, nuts, seeds, and olive oil, which support heart health and provide essential fatty acids.

Practice Portion Control:

Managing portion sizes is essential for weight management. Use smaller plates and bowls to control serving sizes, and listen to your body's hunger and fullness cues. Avoid overeating by eating slowly and mindfully.

Plan Balanced Meals:

Each meal should ideally consist of a balance of macronutrients: carbohydrates, proteins, and fats. Including all three macronutrients helps stabilize blood sugar levels and provides sustained energy throughout the day.

Schedule Regular Meals:

Stick to a consistent meal schedule to avoid excessive snacking or overeating due to hunger. Aim to have three balanced meals a day, with healthy snacks if needed.

Be Mindful of Treats:

Allow yourself occasional treats to satisfy cravings and prevent feelings of deprivation. Moderation is key, and mindful indulgence can help you stay on track without feeling guilty.

Prepare in Advance:

Plan and prepare your meals in advance, if possible, to ensure you have nutritious options readily available. This reduces the temptation to resort to unhealthy choices when time is limited.

Hydration is Key:

Don't forget to stay hydrated throughout the day. Drink plenty of water to support overall health and control appetite.

Monitor and Adjust:

Regularly assess your meal plan and monitor its impact on your weight, energy levels, and overall well-being. Be open to adjustments based on your progress and individual needs.

By creating a balanced and sustainable meal plan, you lay the groundwork for successful weight loss and overall health improvement. Remember that every individual's needs are unique, so it's essential to find a meal plan that suits you best. Embrace this journey as an opportunity to explore new foods, experiment with recipes, and cultivate a healthier relationship with food.

Understanding Macronutrients And Micronutrients

Macronutrients and micronutrients are two essential categories of nutrients that play distinct roles in supporting our overall health and well-being. Each contributes to various bodily functions, and a well-balanced diet should include both to ensure optimal nutrition. Let's explore the differences and roles of macronutrients and micronutrients:

Macronutrients:

Macronutrients are nutrients that our bodies need in large quantities to provide energy and support vital functions. There are three primary macronutrients:

1) Carbohydrates: Carbohydrates are the body's primary source of energy. When consumed, they are broken down into glucose, which our cells use as fuel. Carbohydrates are found in foods like grains, fruits, vegetables, and legumes. Whole, unprocessed carbohydrates, such as whole grains and fruits, are preferred over refined and sugary options.

2) Proteins: Proteins are essential for building and repairing tissues in the body. They also play roles in enzyme production, immune function, and hormone synthesis. Good sources of protein include meat, poultry, fish, eggs, dairy products, legumes, nuts, and seeds.

3) Fats: Fats are another significant source of energy and are crucial for absorbing certain vitamins (fat-soluble vitamins A, D, E, and K). Healthy fats like monounsaturated and polyunsaturated fats are found in foods like avocados, nuts, seeds, and olive oil. Limit intake of saturated and trans fats, often found in processed foods and fatty meats.

Micronutrients:

Micronutrients are nutrients required in smaller quantities, but they are equally vital for proper body function. They include vitamins and minerals, and each one has specific roles in supporting various bodily processes:

1) Vitamins: Vitamins are organic compounds that are essential for normal growth, metabolism, and immune function. They help regulate many biochemical reactions in the body. There are water-soluble vitamins (such as vitamin C and the B-complex vitamins) and fat-soluble vitamins (A, D, E, and K).

2) Minerals: Minerals are inorganic elements critical for various bodily functions, including bone health, nerve function, and fluid balance. Examples of minerals include calcium, iron, magnesium, zinc, and potassium.

Balancing Macronutrients and Micronutrients:

A balanced diet should include an appropriate proportion of macronutrients and a variety of foods to ensure sufficient intake of micronutrients. A diet rich in fruits, vegetables, whole grains, lean proteins, and healthy fats provides the necessary nutrients for optimal health.

Nutrient Density:

Nutrient density refers to the amount of essential nutrients in a food relative to its calorie content. Choosing nutrient-dense foods ensures that you get more essential nutrients per calorie, supporting overall health and weight management.

In conclusion, macronutrients provide energy and support essential bodily functions, while micronutrients are crucial for various biochemical reactions and overall health. A well-balanced diet that includes a variety of nutrient-dense foods ensures that you receive the necessary nutrients for optimal well-being and a healthier life. Remember that individual nutritional needs may vary, so consulting with a registered dietitian can provide personalized guidance for meeting your specific requirements.

Making Healthy Food Choices And Portion Control

Making healthy food choices and practicing portion control are vital components of maintaining a balanced diet and achieving weight loss goals. By being mindful of what and how much you eat, you can support your overall health and well-being. Here are some practical tips to help you make healthier food choices and practice portion control:

Prioritize Nutrient-Dense Foods:
Focus on nutrient-dense foods that provide essential vitamins, minerals, and other nutrients without excessive calories. Choose whole, unprocessed foods like fruits, vegetables, whole grains, lean proteins, nuts, and seeds. These foods offer more nutritional value and are filling, making it easier to maintain a balanced diet.

Read Nutrition Labels:

Become familiar with reading nutrition labels on packaged foods. Pay attention to serving sizes and be mindful of added sugars, unhealthy fats, and excessive sodium. Aim to choose foods with lower amounts of these components to make healthier choices.

Mindful Eating:

Practice mindful eating by being present and attentive during meals. Avoid distractions like electronic devices while eating and savor the flavors and textures of your food. Being mindful of your eating habits can help you recognize true hunger and fullness cues, preventing overeating.

Avoid Emotional Eating:

Be mindful of emotional eating, which occurs when you eat in response to stress, boredom, or other emotions rather than physical hunger. Find alternative ways to cope with emotions, such as engaging in hobbies, exercise, or talking to a friend.

Practice Portion Control:

Be mindful of portion sizes to prevent overeating. Use smaller plates and bowls to help control portions visually. Avoid eating straight from the bag or container, as it can lead to mindless consumption.

Listen to Your Body:

Pay attention to your body's hunger and fullness cues. Eat when you are hungry and stop when you are satisfied, but not overly full. Eating slowly and mindfully can help you recognize these signals more effectively.

Plan Your Meals and Snacks:

Plan your meals and snacks in advance to avoid impulsive choices. This allows you to make healthier options readily available and prevents last-minute unhealthy decisions.

Limit Sugary and Processed Foods:

Reduce your intake of sugary beverages, processed snacks, and foods high in added sugars. Instead, choose whole, natural foods that provide sustained energy and better nutritional value.

Hydration is Key:

Stay hydrated throughout the day by drinking plenty of water. Sometimes, feelings of hunger may be mistaken for thirst. Drinking enough water can help you control your appetite and make healthier food choices.

Allow for Occasional Treats:

Allow yourself occasional treats in moderation. Completely restricting your favorite indulgences can lead to feelings of deprivation and potentially derail your progress. Enjoy treats mindfully and within your overall balanced diet.

Remember that making healthier food choices and practicing portion control are sustainable lifestyle changes. Progress may not be immediate, but with consistent effort and mindful choices, you can develop healthier eating habits that support your long-term health and weight management goals. If needed, seek guidance from a registered dietitian to create a personalized plan that aligns with your individual needs and preferences.

CHAPTER 4: BUILDING HEALTHY EATING HABITS

Building healthy eating habits is essential for long-term success in achieving and maintaining a balanced diet and a healthy weight. This chapter will explore strategies to overcome emotional eating and food cravings, develop mindful eating practices, and incorporate meal prepping and planning for success in your journey towards better eating habits.

Overcoming Emotional Eating And Food Cravings

Emotional eating and food cravings can often lead to unhealthy eating habits, making it challenging to achieve and maintain a balanced diet. However, with mindful strategies and self-awareness, you can effectively overcome these obstacles and develop a healthier relationship with food.

Here are some helpful tips to overcome emotional eating and food cravings:

Identify Triggers:

Take time to recognize the emotions or situations that trigger emotional eating or cravings. Common triggers may include stress, boredom, loneliness, anxiety, or even celebration. By identifying your triggers, you can become more aware of your emotional responses to food and find healthier ways to cope with these emotions.

Practice Mindfulness:

Mindfulness plays a significant role in overcoming emotional eating and food cravings. Before reaching for food, pause and ask yourself if you are physically hungry or if you are seeking comfort or distraction. By being mindful of your hunger and emotions, you can choose more appropriate ways to address your needs.

Find Alternative Coping Strategies:

Instead of turning to food for emotional comfort, explore alternative coping strategies. Engage in activities that bring you joy, such as going for a walk, doing yoga, journaling, practicing deep breathing, or talking to a friend. Finding non-food-related ways to manage emotions helps break the cycle of emotional eating.

Keep a Food and Emotion Journal:

Consider keeping a journal to track your emotions and food choices. Write down what you eat, when you eat, and how you are feeling at the time. This can provide insights into patterns and triggers, enabling you to develop strategies to address emotional eating.

Create a Support System:

Share your journey with friends, family, or a support group. Having a support system can provide encouragement, understanding, and accountability in overcoming emotional eating. Openly discussing your struggles and progress can be empowering and motivate you to make healthier choices.

Avoid Keeping Trigger Foods in the House:

If certain foods consistently trigger cravings, avoid keeping them in your home. Instead, stock your kitchen with nutritious and satisfying alternatives. Having healthier options readily available will make it easier to make positive choices when cravings strike.

Practice Mindful Eating:

When you do choose to eat, practice mindful eating. Slow down, savor each bite, and focus on the taste and texture of the food. By eating mindfully, you can enjoy your meals more fully and recognize feelings of fullness sooner, preventing overeating.

Seek Professional Support:

If emotional eating becomes a persistent issue that interferes with your well-being, consider seeking guidance from a therapist or counselor. They can help you address underlying emotional challenges and develop healthier coping mechanisms.

Remember that overcoming emotional eating and food cravings is a gradual process. Be patient with yourself and celebrate each step forward. By cultivating mindfulness, understanding your triggers, and finding healthier coping strategies, you can successfully break free from emotional eating patterns and develop a healthier and more balanced relationship with food.

Developing Mindful Eating Practices

Mindful eating is a powerful practice that involves being fully present and aware during meals. It allows you to cultivate a healthier and more conscious relationship with food, leading to improved eating habits and overall well-being. Here are some key principles and strategies to help you develop mindful eating practices:

Engage All Your Senses:

Before you start eating, take a moment to appreciate the visual appeal, aroma, and texture of your food. Engaging all your senses allows you to fully experience the meal and enhances the pleasure of eating.

Eliminate Distractions:

Create a calm and distraction-free environment during meals. Turn off electronic devices and avoid multitasking while eating. Focusing solely on your food allows you to connect with the eating experience and recognize your body's hunger and fullness cues.

Eat Slowly and Chew Thoroughly:

Chew your food slowly and thoroughly. Eating slowly helps with digestion and allows your brain to register feelings of satiety, preventing overeating. Put your utensils down between bites to savor each mouthful.

Listen to Your Body's Hunger Cues:

Pay attention to your body's signals of hunger and fullness. Eat when you are physically hungry, and stop when you feel satisfied, but not overly full. Listening to your body's cues helps you avoid mindless eating and promotes a more balanced intake of food.

Be Non-Judgmental:

Adopt a non-judgmental attitude towards your eating habits. Avoid labeling foods as "good" or "bad." Instead, focus on making mindful choices that nourish your body and bring enjoyment to your meals.

Notice Emotional Eating Triggers:

Mindful eating involves being aware of emotional eating triggers. When you notice the desire to eat arising from emotions rather than hunger, pause and acknowledge the emotions without judgment. Explore alternative coping mechanisms for addressing emotional needs.

Practice Gratitude:

Take a moment to express gratitude for the food you are about to eat and the effort that went into preparing it. Gratitude enhances the eating experience and encourages a positive attitude towards food.

Portion Control:

Be mindful of portion sizes and avoid overeating. Use smaller plates and serve appropriate portions to prevent the temptation to consume more than your body needs.

Enjoy Balanced Meals:
Create balanced meals that include a variety of nutrient-dense foods. Include a mix of carbohydrates, proteins, healthy fats, and plenty of fruits and vegetables in your meals to ensure nutritional adequacy.

Forgive Yourself for Mistakes:
Mindful eating is a journey, and it's natural to have moments of mindless eating or lapses. If you find yourself overeating or making less mindful choices, forgive yourself and use it as a learning opportunity to enhance your mindful eating practice moving forward.

In conclusion, developing mindful eating practices requires patience, self-compassion, and consistent effort. By embracing the principles of mindfulness, being present during meals, and listening to your body's signals, you can develop a healthier and more mindful approach to eating. Mindful eating fosters a deeper appreciation for food and nourishment, leading to improved eating habits and greater overall well-being.

Meal Prepping And Planning For Success

Meal prepping and planning are essential strategies for achieving weight loss success. By preparing nutritious meals in advance and thoughtfully organizing your eating schedule, you can stay on track with your health goals and make healthier choices throughout the day. Here are some valuable tips for incorporating meal prepping and planning into your weight loss journey:

Plan Your Meals Ahead of Time:

Create a weekly meal plan that includes a variety of balanced and nutritious meals. Planning your meals in advance allows you to make healthier choices, reduces the temptation to indulge in less nutritious options, and helps you stay organized.

Include a Mix of Macronutrients:

Ensure that your meals consist of a mix of macronutrients - carbohydrates, proteins, and healthy fats. This combination keeps you feeling full and satisfied while supporting your body's nutritional needs.

Opt for Nutrient-Dense Foods:

Choose nutrient-dense foods such as fruits, vegetables, whole grains, lean proteins, and healthy fats. These foods are rich in vitamins, minerals, and fiber, providing essential nutrients without excess calories.

Prepare Portion-Controlled Meals:
Use portion-controlled containers or dividers to create balanced and appropriate serving sizes. Portion control helps you manage calorie intake and prevents overeating.

Batch Cooking:
Cook large quantities of certain meals at once and store them in individual portions for the week. Batch cooking saves time and ensures that you always have healthy options available.

Stock Healthy Snacks:
Prepare and portion healthy snacks like cut-up fruits, raw nuts, or vegetable sticks. Having these snacks readily available prevents you from reaching for less nutritious options when hunger strikes.

Organize a Weekly Grocery List:
Based on your meal plan, create a weekly grocery list and stick to it while shopping. This prevents impulse purchases

and ensures you have all the ingredients needed for your prepped meals.

Prep Ingredients in Advance:

Wash, chop, and prepare ingredients ahead of time to streamline meal preparation during busy days. Having ingredients ready to use makes cooking quicker and more convenient.

Use Time-Saving Kitchen Tools:

Consider investing in time-saving kitchen tools like a slow cooker, pressure cooker, or blender. These appliances make meal preparation easier and more efficient.

Stay Consistent:

Consistency is key to successful weight loss. Stick to your meal prepping and planning routine, and make it a regular part of your lifestyle. Consistency helps build healthy habits that contribute to long-term success.

Allow Flexibility:

While meal prepping and planning can be structured, allow room for flexibility. Embrace occasional changes to your schedule or spontaneous dining-out experiences without feeling guilty. Flexibility ensures that your meal prepping remains sustainable and adaptable to different situations.

By incorporating meal prepping and planning into your weight loss journey, you create a supportive environment that promotes healthier choices and consistency. It saves time, reduces stress, and empowers you to make mindful eating decisions, ultimately contributing to your weight loss success and improved overall well-being.

.

CHAPTER 5: THE POWER OF PHYSICAL ACTIVITY

Physical activity is a key component of any successful weight loss journey. This chapter explores the significance of finding enjoyable and effective exercise routines, incorporating physical activity into a busy lifestyle, and the multiple benefits of regular exercise beyond weight loss.

Finding Enjoyable And Effective Exercise Routines

Discovering exercise routines that are both enjoyable and effective is crucial for maintaining motivation and consistency in your fitness journey. When you enjoy your workouts, you are more likely to stick with them, leading to better results and an overall positive exercise experience. Here are some tips to help you find enjoyable and effective exercise routines:

Try Different Activities:

Experiment with a variety of exercises to find what you genuinely enjoy. There are numerous options available, such as running, swimming, cycling, dancing, yoga, weightlifting, martial arts, and group fitness classes. Be open to trying new activities and see which ones resonate with you the most.

Consider Your Interests:

Incorporate exercises that align with your interests and passions. If you enjoy being outdoors, consider hiking or trail running. If you prefer social interactions, join a sports team or group exercise class. When you engage in activities that excite you, working out becomes more fun and fulfilling.

Set Clear Goals:

Define your fitness goals and choose exercises that align with them. For example, if your goal is to improve cardiovascular health, focus on aerobic activities like jogging or cycling. If you want to build strength and muscle, incorporate resistance training into your routine.

Mix It Up:

Avoid monotony by including a mix of activities in your routine. Variety not only keeps things interesting but also helps target different muscle groups and prevent overuse injuries. Alternating between cardio, strength training, flexibility exercises, and other forms of movement can provide a well-rounded fitness experience.

Make It Social:

Work out with friends, family, or join group fitness classes to add a social element to your exercise routine. Socializing while exercising can boost motivation, accountability, and make workouts more enjoyable.

Use Technology:

Embrace fitness apps or online platforms that offer guided workouts, challenges, or interactive features. These tools can add an element of excitement and novelty to your routine.

Listen to Your Body:

Pay attention to how your body responds to different exercises. If a particular activity causes discomfort or doesn't feel right, don't be afraid to try something else. Finding exercises that are comfortable and enjoyable will make your fitness journey more sustainable.

Track Your Progress:

Document your fitness journey, noting how you feel after each workout and any improvements you notice over time. Tracking your progress can be highly motivating and help you celebrate your achievements.

Incorporate Music or Podcasts:

Listening to your favorite music or podcasts during workouts can make the experience more enjoyable and distract you from any perceived exertion.

Make It a Habit:

Consistency is key to finding enjoyment and seeing results from your exercise routine. Make physical activity a regular part of your daily or weekly schedule to develop a habit that becomes second nature.

Remember that everyone's preferences and interests are different, so take the time to explore and find the exercise routines that bring you joy and satisfaction. Ultimately, finding enjoyable and effective exercise routines will not only enhance your fitness journey but also contribute to your overall health and well-being.

Incorporating Physical Activity Into A Busy Lifestyle

Incorporating physical activity into a busy lifestyle can be challenging, but it is essential for maintaining overall health and well-being. By finding creative ways to move your body throughout the day, you can stay active even amidst a hectic schedule. Here are some strategies to help you incorporate physical activity into your busy lifestyle:

Schedule Exercise Time:

Treat physical activity as a priority and schedule it into your daily agenda. Block out specific time slots for workouts, just as you would for other important appointments. Consistency in scheduling helps establish exercise as a regular part of your routine.

Opt for Shorter Workouts:

If time is limited, focus on shorter, high-intensity workouts. High-intensity interval training (HIIT) or circuit training can be effective in a shorter time frame and provide similar benefits to longer workouts.

Break Up Sedentary Behavior:

Incorporate movement breaks during prolonged periods of sitting. Set reminders to stand up, stretch, or walk around for a few minutes every hour. These mini-breaks can improve circulation and help prevent stiffness.

Use Active Transportation:

Whenever possible, choose active transportation options. Walk or bike to work, school, or nearby errands instead of driving. This not only adds physical activity to your day but also reduces your carbon footprint.

Make It a Family Affair:

If you have family members with busy schedules, involve them in physical activities. Go for a family walk after dinner or participate in active outings on the weekends. This fosters a healthy lifestyle for everyone and encourages bonding.

Utilize Break Times:

During work breaks, lunch breaks, or other downtime, find opportunities to move. Take a brisk walk around your office building, climb a few flights of stairs, or do some stretching exercises to stay active throughout the day.

Choose Activities You Enjoy:

Incorporate physical activities that you genuinely enjoy. When you look forward to an activity, it becomes easier to make time for it in your busy schedule. Whether it's dancing, playing a sport, or gardening, finding pleasure in the activity keeps you motivated.

Combine Work and Exercise:

If possible, combine work-related tasks with physical activity. Consider walking meetings, using a standing desk, or doing some desk exercises to keep your body active while getting work done.

Be Efficient with Time:

Maximize your workout time by choosing exercises that target multiple muscle groups simultaneously. Compound movements like squats, lunges, and push-ups work several muscles at once, saving time while providing an effective workout.

Prioritize Rest and Recovery:

Balancing a busy lifestyle with physical activity requires proper rest and recovery. Listen to your body and ensure you get enough sleep to support your energy levels and overall well-being.

In conclusion, incorporating physical activity into a busy lifestyle is achievable with planning, creativity, and consistency. By making small changes to your daily habits and finding ways to move your body throughout the day, you can reap the benefits of regular exercise without overwhelming your schedule. Remember that every bit of activity counts, and even short bursts of movement can make a positive impact on your health and fitness.

Benefits Of Regular Exercise Beyond Weight Loss

Regular exercise offers a myriad of benefits beyond weight loss, making it a crucial component of a healthy lifestyle. Whether you are looking to maintain your current weight or have already achieved your weight loss goals, incorporating physical activity into your routine can significantly enhance your overall well-being. Here are some of the key benefits of regular exercise:

Improved Cardiovascular Health:
Engaging in regular aerobic exercises, such as running, swimming, or cycling, improves cardiovascular health. Exercise strengthens the heart, increases blood flow, and helps lower blood pressure, reducing the risk of heart disease and stroke.

Enhanced Mental Health:
Physical activity has a powerful impact on mental health and well-being. Regular exercise triggers the release of endorphins, neurotransmitters that elevate mood and reduce stress and anxiety. It can also help alleviate symptoms of depression and improve cognitive function.

Increased Energy and Endurance:

Consistent physical activity boosts energy levels and endurance. Regular exercise improves oxygen and nutrient delivery to the muscles, making daily tasks feel less tiring and providing greater stamina for physical activities.

Better Sleep Quality:

Regular exercise promotes better sleep patterns and improves sleep quality. People who engage in physical activity tend to fall asleep faster, experience deeper sleep, and wake up feeling more refreshed.

Strengthened Muscles and Bones:

Strength training exercises, such as weightlifting or resistance training, build and tone muscles while promoting bone health. Regular resistance training can help reduce the risk of age-related muscle loss and osteoporosis.

Enhanced Flexibility and Balance:

Activities like yoga and stretching exercises improve flexibility, balance, and joint mobility. This can help prevent injuries and improve overall physical performance.

Reduced Risk of Chronic Diseases:

Regular exercise lowers the risk of chronic conditions such as type 2 diabetes, certain cancers, and metabolic disorders. It can also help manage existing conditions and improve overall health outcomes.

Boosted Immune System:
Regular moderate-intensity exercise strengthens the immune system, reducing the risk of infections and illnesses. However, excessive exercise without adequate recovery may weaken the immune system.

Improved Digestive Health:
Physical activity can aid in promoting healthy digestion and regulating bowel movements. It can help prevent constipation and improve gastrointestinal function.

Increased Longevity:
Numerous studies have shown that regular exercise is associated with increased life expectancy. Engaging in physical activity consistently can add years to your life and enhance the quality of those years.

Enhanced Self-Esteem and Body Image:
Exercise has the potential to improve self-esteem and body image. Achieving fitness goals and feeling stronger and more

confident in your body can positively impact self-perception.

In conclusion, regular exercise is a powerful tool for promoting overall health and well-being. Beyond weight loss, physical activity offers a wide range of benefits, including improved cardiovascular health, enhanced mental well-being, increased energy levels, and reduced risk of chronic diseases. Whether you're already at a healthy weight or still on your weight loss journey, incorporating regular exercise into your lifestyle can significantly contribute to a happier, healthier, and more vibrant life.

CHAPTER 6: CREATING A SUPPORTIVE ENVIRONMENT

Creating a supportive environment is essential for maintaining motivation, staying on track with your goals, and fostering a positive mindset throughout your health and wellness journey. This chapter explores the importance of building a positive and encouraging support system, managing stress and emotional well-being, and surrounding yourself with like-minded individuals who share your health aspirations.

Building A Positive And Encouraging Support System

Building a positive and encouraging support system is crucial for achieving success in various aspects of life, including health and well-being. A strong support system can provide motivation, guidance, and emotional reinforcement, helping you stay focused on your goals and overcome challenges. Here are some key steps to build a positive and encouraging support system:

Identify Supportive Individuals:

Start by identifying people in your life who genuinely care about your well-being and are willing to support you on your journey. This could include family members, friends, colleagues, or mentors who share your values or have similar health goals.

Communicate Your Goals:

Share your health and wellness goals with your support network. By articulating your aspirations, you invite them to be part of your journey and understand the significance of their encouragement.

Seek Empathy and Understanding:

Look for individuals who can empathize with your struggles and challenges. Having someone who understands what you're going through and can provide empathy and encouragement can make a significant difference in your motivation and perseverance.

Set Boundaries:

Ensure that your support system respects your boundaries and provides encouragement rather than judgment. Healthy support involves understanding that everyone's journey is unique and that progress may come at different paces.

Join Supportive Communities:

Consider joining local or online support groups that align with your health and wellness interests. Engaging with like-minded individuals can foster a sense of camaraderie and provide additional perspectives and insights.

Share Progress and Celebrate Achievements:

Regularly update your support system on your progress and celebrate your achievements together. Celebrating milestones, no matter how small, reinforces your dedication and inspires continued effort.

Be Open to Feedback:

Be open to constructive feedback from your support system. Sometimes, they may provide valuable insights, suggestions, or alternative approaches that can help you overcome obstacles and enhance your well-being journey.

Offer Support in Return:

Support is a two-way street. Be willing to reciprocate and provide encouragement to your support system when they need it. Offering support and being there for others can strengthen the bond and create a mutually beneficial relationship.

Surround Yourself with Positive Influence:
Seek out individuals who radiate positivity and optimism. Positive influences can uplift your spirits, boost your confidence, and help you maintain a positive outlook on your health and life goals.

Be Patient and Understanding:
Remember that building a strong support system takes time and effort. Be patient and understanding, and be willing to nurture these relationships to foster an encouraging environment.

In conclusion, a positive and encouraging support system is a valuable asset in achieving your health and wellness objectives. By identifying supportive individuals, communicating your goals, and being open to feedback, you create a network of people who inspire and motivate you on your journey. Cultivating these positive relationships will not only benefit your well-being but also contribute to a more fulfilling and enjoyable life overall.

Managing Stress And Emotional Well-Being

Managing stress and emotional well-being is crucial for maintaining overall health and happiness. In today's fast-paced world, stress can be a common occurrence, but learning to manage it effectively is essential for leading a balanced and fulfilling life. Here are some strategies to help you manage stress and nurture your emotional well-being:

Identify Stress Triggers:

Start by identifying the sources of stress in your life. Recognize the situations, events, or people that tend to cause stress and take note of how you react to them. Understanding your stress triggers can help you develop coping strategies.

Practice Mindfulness and Meditation:

Mindfulness and meditation are powerful tools for managing stress and promoting emotional well-being. These practices help you stay present in the moment, cultivate self-awareness, and reduce anxiety and racing thoughts.

Engage in Regular Physical Activity:

Regular exercise is an excellent way to reduce stress and improve emotional well-being. Physical activity releases endorphins, which act as natural mood lifters, helping you feel more relaxed and content.

Prioritize Self-Care:

Make time for self-care activities that bring you joy and relaxation. This can include spending time in nature, reading, journaling, or engaging in hobbies you love. Taking care of yourself emotionally is essential for overall well-being.

Set Realistic Goals and Prioritize Tasks:
Set achievable goals and prioritize tasks to avoid feeling overwhelmed. Break larger tasks into smaller, manageable steps, and focus on one thing at a time. This approach can help reduce stress and increase productivity.

Practice Deep Breathing Techniques:
Deep breathing exercises can help calm the nervous system and reduce stress. Take slow, deep breaths, inhaling deeply through your nose and exhaling slowly through your mouth. Repeat several times whenever you feel stressed.

Develop Healthy Coping Mechanisms:
Avoid using unhealthy coping mechanisms, such as excessive alcohol consumption or emotional eating, to deal with stress. Instead, find healthier ways to cope, such as talking to a friend, engaging in creative outlets, or seeking professional help.

Maintain a Support System:

Having a strong support system can provide emotional comfort and reduce stress. Talk to friends or family members about your feelings, and seek their support when needed. Sometimes, simply expressing your emotions can be cathartic.

Limit Exposure to Stressors:

Identify stressors that are within your control and take steps to limit your exposure to them. Set boundaries with work, social commitments, or digital devices to create a more balanced and stress-free environment.

Seek Professional Help if Needed:

If stress becomes overwhelming or persistent, consider seeking support from a therapist or counselor. Professional help can provide valuable guidance and strategies to manage stress and improve emotional well-being.

In conclusion, managing stress and nurturing your emotional well-being is essential for leading a healthy and fulfilling life. By adopting stress-reducing practices, prioritizing self-care, and seeking support when needed, you can create a more balanced and resilient mindset. Remember that everyone experiences stress, and it's okay to seek help and support in managing it. Taking care of your emotional well-being will positively impact your overall health and empower you to navigate life's challenges with greater resilience and peace of mind.

Surrounding Yourself With Like-Minded Individuals

Surrounding yourself with like-minded individuals can have a profound impact on your personal growth, well-being, and success. Like-minded people share similar interests, values, and goals, creating a supportive and encouraging environment that fosters mutual growth and understanding. Here are some benefits and strategies for surrounding yourself with like-minded individuals:

Benefits of Being Around Like-Minded Individuals:

1. Shared Understanding: Like-minded individuals understand and relate to your experiences, challenges, and aspirations. This shared understanding creates a sense of camaraderie and validation.

2. Motivation and Encouragement: Being around people who share similar goals can be highly motivating. You can inspire each other to stay focused, overcome obstacles, and celebrate achievements together.

3. Positive Influence: Surrounding yourself with like-minded individuals who have a positive outlook on life can influence your mindset and foster optimism and resilience.

4. Enhanced Learning and Growth: Engaging with people who have different perspectives and knowledge can broaden your understanding and promote personal growth.

5. Networking Opportunities: Being part of a like-minded community can provide networking opportunities and connections that can be valuable in various aspects of life.

Strategies for Surrounding Yourself with Like-Minded Individuals:

Join Communities or Clubs: Seek out local or online communities, clubs, or organizations that align with your interests and values. Whether it's a fitness group, book club, or professional association, being part of a community with shared interests can be enriching.

Attend Events and Workshops: Participate in events, workshops, or seminars that focus on subjects you are passionate about. These gatherings are great opportunities to connect with like-minded individuals.

Utilize Social Media: Engage with social media platforms that cater to your interests and goals. Join groups or follow accounts that resonate with your passions, and participate in meaningful discussions.

Attend Meetups or Networking Events: Attend meetups or networking events in your area to connect with people who share similar interests or career aspirations.

Be Open and Approachable: Be open to meeting new people and engaging in conversations. Approach others with a friendly demeanor and a willingness to learn from their experiences.

Share Your Interests and Goals: Communicate your interests and goals with others. By expressing your passions, you attract like-minded individuals who share your enthusiasm.

Be Supportive and Empathetic: Cultivate a supportive and empathetic attitude towards others. Show genuine interest in their journeys and offer encouragement and assistance when needed.

Embrace Diversity: While seeking like-minded individuals, also embrace diversity and different perspectives. Being open to learning from people with varied backgrounds enriches your understanding and promotes personal growth.

Share Your Knowledge and Skills: Offer your knowledge and skills to others in your community. Being a helpful and supportive member fosters a sense of belonging and strengthens the bond within the group.

Nurture Relationships: Building relationships takes time and effort. Nurture your connections with like-minded individuals by staying engaged, being present, and offering your support.

In conclusion, surrounding yourself with like-minded individuals can significantly enhance your personal growth, well-being, and success. Being part of a supportive community that shares your interests and values provides encouragement, motivation, and a sense of belonging. Embrace opportunities to connect with like-minded people, and in return, contribute positively to the growth and well-being of those around you. Together, you can create a thriving environment that uplifts each member and empowers everyone to reach their full potential.

CHAPTER 7: LIFESTYLE CHANGES FOR LASTING RESULTS

In the pursuit of lasting weight loss results, it's essential to embrace lifestyle changes that become a sustainable part of your daily routine. This chapter delves into integrating healthy habits into daily life, strategies for maintaining weight loss over the long term, and adapting to setbacks while staying motivated on your weight loss journey.

Integrating Healthy Habits Into Daily Life

Integrating healthy habits into daily life is essential for achieving lasting well-being and improved overall health. By making healthy choices a natural part of your routine, you create a sustainable lifestyle that supports your physical, mental, and emotional well-being. Here are some strategies to help you integrate healthy habits into your daily life:

Start Small:
Begin by incorporating small, manageable changes into your daily routine. Focus on one or two healthy habits at a time, such as drinking more water or adding a serving of vegetables to your meals. Starting small allows you to build

momentum and increases the likelihood of long-term success.

Create a Daily Routine:

Establish a daily schedule that includes time for healthy habits. Allocate specific time slots for exercise, meal preparation, relaxation, and other activities that contribute to your well-being. A consistent routine makes it easier to stick to healthy habits.

Set Realistic Goals:

Set achievable and realistic health goals that align with your lifestyle and preferences. Avoid setting overly ambitious targets that might become overwhelming. Celebrate your progress, no matter how small, and use it as motivation to keep going.

Make Healthy Eating Convenient:

Stock your pantry and fridge with nutritious foods and snacks. Plan your meals in advance and prep ingredients when possible. Having healthy options readily available makes it easier to resist unhealthy temptations.

Find Exercise You Enjoy:

Explore various forms of physical activity to find what you genuinely enjoy. Whether it's dancing, hiking, cycling, or practicing yoga, engaging in activities you love increases your chances of sticking to an exercise routine.

Incorporate Movement Throughout the Day:
Look for opportunities to move throughout your day, even if you have a sedentary job. Take short breaks to stretch or walk, use the stairs instead of the elevator, or do a quick workout during lunch breaks.

Practice Mindful Eating:
Pay attention to your hunger and fullness cues during meals. Avoid distractions like TV or smartphones while eating and savor the flavors and textures of your food. Mindful eating can help prevent overeating and improve digestion.

Prioritize Sleep:
Establish a consistent sleep schedule to ensure you get enough rest each night. Make your sleep environment comfortable and free of distractions to promote restful sleep.

Manage Stress:

Incorporate stress-reducing practices like meditation, deep breathing, or spending time in nature. Managing stress is crucial for overall well-being and can positively impact your eating habits and sleep quality.

Stay Hydrated:

Keep a water bottle with you throughout the day and make it a habit to drink water regularly. Staying hydrated supports your body's functions and can help control hunger.

Seek Social Support:

Engage with friends, family, or colleagues who share your interest in healthy living. Surrounding yourself with supportive individuals can make adopting healthy habits more enjoyable and sustainable.

Be Patient and Kind to Yourself:

Remember that forming new habits takes time, and it's normal to face challenges along the way. Be patient with yourself and avoid self-criticism. Embrace each day as an opportunity to make progress toward a healthier lifestyle.

In conclusion, integrating healthy habits into daily life is a gradual and rewarding process. By starting small, setting realistic goals, and prioritizing self-care, you can create a lifestyle that supports your overall health and well-being. Embrace the journey of making positive changes and celebrate each step toward a healthier and more fulfilling life.

Strategies For Maintaining Weight Loss Over The Long Term

Maintaining weight loss over the long term can be just as challenging as losing the weight in the first place. To ensure lasting success, it's crucial to implement strategies that support continued progress and prevent relapses. Here are some effective strategies for maintaining weight loss over the long term:

Establish Realistic Goals:
Set realistic and sustainable weight maintenance goals. Avoid extreme diets or unrealistic expectations that are difficult to maintain in the long run. Aim for a gradual, steady approach to weight maintenance.

Embrace a Balanced Diet:
Continue to follow a balanced and nutritious diet that includes a variety of foods from all food groups. Avoid

restrictive diets and focus on nourishing your body with wholesome, satisfying meals.

Monitor Your Progress:

Regularly track your weight, food intake, and physical activity to stay aware of your progress. Monitoring helps you identify potential challenges early on and allows you to make necessary adjustments to maintain your weight loss.

Stay Physically Active:

Maintain a consistent exercise routine that you enjoy. Regular physical activity not only supports weight maintenance but also provides numerous health benefits for your body and mind.

Practice Mindful Eating:

Continue to practice mindful eating by paying attention to hunger and fullness cues, avoiding emotional eating, and savoring your meals. Mindful eating helps you make conscious food choices and prevents overeating.

Plan Your Meals:

Plan your meals and snacks in advance to avoid impulsive and unhealthy choices. Meal planning can help you make nutritious and portion-controlled meals, reducing the likelihood of weight regain.

Manage Stress:

Stress can trigger emotional eating and undermine weight maintenance efforts. Employ stress management techniques, such as meditation, yoga, or deep breathing exercises, to cope with stress effectively.

Prioritize Sleep:

Ensure you get enough quality sleep each night. Adequate sleep supports overall well-being and helps regulate hunger hormones, reducing the risk of weight gain.

Surround Yourself with Supportive People:

Maintain connections with supportive friends, family members, or weight loss support groups. Having a positive and encouraging support system can significantly impact your ability to maintain weight loss.

Monitor Eating Triggers:

Be mindful of eating triggers, such as boredom, stress, or social situations. Develop alternative coping mechanisms to deal with emotions or situations that might lead to overeating.

Limit Highly Processed Foods:

Reduce your consumption of highly processed foods and sugary beverages. These items often provide empty calories and can hinder your weight maintenance efforts.

Celebrate Non-Scale Victories:

Recognize and celebrate non-scale victories, such as increased energy, improved fitness levels, or enhanced confidence. Acknowledging these achievements reinforces your commitment to a healthy lifestyle.

Seek Professional Support:

If you encounter challenges in maintaining your weight loss, consider seeking guidance from a registered dietitian or a weight loss counselor. They can provide personalized strategies and motivation.

Embrace a Positive Mindset:

Maintain a positive attitude and avoid self-criticism. Embrace the journey of weight maintenance as a lifelong commitment to your health and well-being.

In conclusion, maintaining weight loss over the long term requires dedication, consistency, and a focus on sustainable lifestyle changes. By implementing these strategies and staying mindful of your health and well-being, you can enjoy the rewards of lasting weight maintenance and improved overall health. Remember that maintaining weight loss is an ongoing process, and each day is an opportunity to continue making positive choices for a healthier and happier life.

Adapting To Setbacks And Staying Motivated

Adapting to setbacks and staying motivated is a crucial aspect of any journey, including weight loss. Setbacks are a natural part of life, and how you respond to them can make a significant difference in your success. Here are some strategies to help you navigate setbacks and maintain motivation on your weight loss journey:

Embrace a Growth Mindset:
View setbacks as opportunities for learning and growth rather than failures. Understand that setbacks are normal and can provide valuable insights into areas that need improvement.

Analyze the Setback:
Take some time to reflect on the setback and identify the factors that contributed to it. Understanding the root causes

can help you develop strategies to prevent similar setbacks in the future.

Setbacks ≠ Failure:

Remind yourself that a setback does not define your overall progress or success. It's a temporary obstacle that you can overcome with determination and perseverance.

Practice Self-Compassion:

Be kind to yourself during setbacks and avoid self-criticism. Treat yourself with the same kindness and understanding that you would offer to a friend facing a similar situation.

Revisit Your Goals:

Reconnect with your long-term goals and the reasons why you started your weight loss journey. Visualize your desired outcomes to renew your motivation and commitment.

Focus on Non-Scale Victories:

Celebrate non-scale victories, such as improved energy levels, increased stamina, or positive changes in your mood. Acknowledging these achievements can boost your confidence and motivation.

Seek Support:

Reach out to your support system, such as friends, family, or a weight loss group, during challenging times. Sharing your setbacks and seeking encouragement can provide emotional reinforcement.

Break Goals into Smaller Steps:

If your goals feel overwhelming, break them into smaller, achievable steps. Celebrate each milestone you reach, as it demonstrates progress towards your ultimate objective.

Practice Positive Self-Talk:

Replace negative thoughts with positive affirmations. Encourage yourself, focus on your strengths, and remind yourself of past successes to maintain a positive mindset.

Find New Inspiration:

Seek inspiration from success stories, motivational quotes, or role models who have achieved similar goals. Their stories can remind you that setbacks are temporary and success is possible.

Create a Plan for Future Setbacks:

Prepare yourself for future setbacks by creating a contingency plan. Identify potential challenges and develop strategies to handle them effectively.

Reframe Setbacks as Learning Opportunities:
Rather than viewing setbacks as failures, see them as learning opportunities. Analyze what went wrong and use that knowledge to make better choices moving forward.

Stay Present:
Focus on the present moment and take things one step at a time. Dwelling on past setbacks or worrying about future challenges can sap your motivation. Stay grounded in the here and now.

Celebrate Resilience:
Recognize your resilience in overcoming setbacks and staying committed to your goals. Each time you bounce back, you demonstrate strength and determination.

In conclusion, setbacks are a natural part of any journey, including weight loss. Adapting to setbacks and staying motivated requires a positive mindset, self-compassion, and a willingness to learn and grow. Remember that progress is not always linear, and setbacks do not define your overall success. Embrace the challenges as opportunities for growth, stay focused on your long-term goals, and draw support from those around you. With determination and resilience, you can navigate setbacks and continue moving forward on your weight loss journey.

Chapter 8: Addressing Weight Loss Plateaus

Weight loss plateaus are common and can be frustrating, but they are a natural part of the weight loss process. This chapter explores the reasons for weight loss plateaus, provides tips and tricks for breaking through them, and offers guidance to avoid common pitfalls that can hinder progress.

Understanding Common Reasons For Weight Loss Plateaus

Understanding the common reasons for weight loss plateaus is essential for effectively addressing and overcoming them. Plateaus occur when your weight loss stalls, and it can be frustrating and demotivating. However, recognizing the underlying factors can help you make necessary adjustments and continue making progress toward your weight loss goals. Here are some common reasons for weight loss plateaus:

Metabolic Adaptation: When you lose weight, your body may adjust its metabolic rate to conserve energy. As a result, your calorie expenditure decreases, and weight loss slows down.

Loss of Muscle Mass: During weight loss, there's a risk of losing both fat and muscle mass. Muscle loss can lower your metabolic rate, making it harder to continue losing weight.

Inadequate Calorie Deficit: As you lose weight, your calorie needs decrease because there is less of you to maintain. If you don't adjust your calorie intake accordingly, the calorie deficit becomes smaller, and weight loss slows down.

Water Retention: Fluctuations in water retention can mask fat loss on the scale, making it appear as though you've hit a plateau when, in reality, you're still making progress.

Hormonal Factors: Hormonal changes can influence appetite, fat storage, and energy expenditure. Hormonal imbalances or changes may affect your weight loss rate.

Reduced Non-Exercise Activity Thermogenesis (NEAT): During weight loss, you may subconsciously reduce your daily physical activities, such as fidgeting or walking, which contributes to a decrease in overall calorie expenditure.

Inconsistent Exercise Routine: Your body can adapt to repetitive exercise routines, causing the calorie burn to become less efficient. Changing up your workouts can help break through plateaus.

Mindless Eating: Eating without being aware of portion sizes or consuming high-calorie foods can hinder weight loss progress.

Stress and Cortisol Levels: Chronic stress can elevate cortisol levels, which may lead to increased fat storage, especially in the abdominal area.

Insufficient Sleep: Poor sleep habits can disrupt hormone levels, affecting appetite regulation and metabolism.

Recognizing these common reasons for weight loss plateaus can empower you to make informed choices to overcome them. It's important to remember that weight loss is not always linear, and plateaus are a natural part of the process. Be patient, stay consistent with your healthy habits, and be open to making necessary adjustments to your approach.

Consulting with a healthcare professional or a registered dietitian can also provide personalized guidance and support to navigate weight loss plateaus successfully.

Tips And Tricks For Breaking Through Plateaus

Breaking through weight loss plateaus requires a strategic approach to jumpstart your progress and continue moving toward your goals. Here are some effective tips and tricks to help you break through weight loss plateaus:

Reassess Your Caloric Intake: Evaluate your current calorie intake and adjust it to match your current weight. As you lose weight, your calorie needs decrease, so it's essential to recalculate your calorie deficit for continued progress.

Mix Up Your Exercise Routine: Vary your exercise routine to challenge your body and prevent adaptation. Incorporate new exercises, change the intensity, or try different workout formats to keep your body guessing.

Strength Training: Incorporate strength training exercises into your routine to build lean muscle mass. Muscle burns more calories at rest than fat, which can help increase your metabolic rate.

Increase Protein Intake: Ensure you're consuming enough protein to support muscle preservation during weight loss. Protein helps you feel fuller and may aid in maintaining lean muscle mass.

Practice Intermittent Fasting: Intermittent fasting can help with breaking plateaus by giving your body a chance to reset and promoting fat burning during the fasting period.

Be Mindful of Portion Sizes: Pay attention to portion sizes, as even healthy foods can contribute to weight gain if consumed in excess. Consider using smaller plates and bowls to manage portion control.

Try Carb Cycling: Alternating between higher and lower carbohydrate intake on different days can help prevent metabolic adaptation and stimulate fat loss.

Monitor Your Water Intake: Ensure you're adequately hydrated, as dehydration can impact your body's ability to burn fat efficiently.

Practice High-Intensity Interval Training (HIIT):
HIIT workouts involve short bursts of intense exercise followed by periods of rest. This can elevate your calorie burn and boost metabolism post-workout.

Manage Stress: High levels of stress can hinder weight loss progress. Engage in stress-reduction techniques such as meditation, yoga, or deep breathing exercises.

Prioritize Sleep: Aim for 7-9 hours of quality sleep each night. Poor sleep can disrupt hormones related to appetite regulation and fat storage.

Review Hidden Calories: Be mindful of hidden calories in sauces, dressings, and beverages. These extra calories can add up and stall your weight loss progress.

Be Patient and Persistent: Breaking through plateaus takes time and consistency. Avoid becoming discouraged and stay committed to your healthy habits.

Seek Support: Talk to friends, family, or a healthcare professional about your weight loss journey. Having a support system can provide encouragement and guidance during plateaus.

Remember that weight loss plateaus are normal and part of the process. Celebrate your progress, focus on the positive changes in your body and lifestyle, and trust that by incorporating these tips and tricks, you'll eventually break through the plateau and continue your journey to a healthier you.

Avoiding Common Pitfalls That Can Hinder Progress

Avoiding common pitfalls that can hinder progress is essential to maintain consistency and continue making strides toward your weight loss goals. Identifying and overcoming these obstacles can significantly impact your success. Here are some common pitfalls to avoid:

Over-Restrictive Diets: Extremely restrictive diets are challenging to sustain and may lead to nutrient deficiencies. Choose a balanced and sustainable eating plan that includes a variety of foods from all food groups.

Mindlcss Eating: Eating without being aware of portion sizes or consuming high-calorie foods can hinder weight loss progress. Be mindful of what and how much you eat.

Emotional Eating: Using food as a way to cope with emotions or stress can lead to overeating and hinder weight loss. Find alternative coping mechanisms such as engaging in hobbies, talking to a friend, or practicing relaxation techniques.

Ignoring Liquid Calories: Be mindful of the calories in beverages such as sugary drinks, alcoholic beverages, and high-calorie coffee drinks. These liquid calories can add up quickly and impede weight loss.

Skipping Meals: Skipping meals can lead to overeating later in the day and disrupt your metabolism. Stick to regular, balanced meals and snacks to maintain steady energy levels.

Lack of Sleep: Inadequate sleep can disrupt hormones related to appetite regulation and fat storage. Aim for 7-9 hours of quality sleep each night to support weight loss efforts.

Inconsistent Exercise Routine: Maintaining a consistent exercise routine is crucial for weight loss. Avoid skipping workouts or being inconsistent with your physical activity.

Impatience and Unrealistic Expectations: Weight loss takes time and effort. Avoid expecting rapid results and recognize that progress may be gradual.

Focusing Solely on the Scale: Weight fluctuates naturally due to factors like water retention and hormonal changes. Don't solely rely on the scale for progress assessment; consider other indicators such as improved fitness levels, clothing fit, and measurements.

Comparing Yourself to Others: Each individual's weight loss journey is unique. Avoid comparing your progress to others and focus on your own achievements.

Neglecting Self-Care: Prioritize self-care and manage stress effectively. Chronic stress can hinder weight loss progress and overall well-being.

All-or-Nothing Mindset: Avoid thinking that one small setback derails all your efforts. Acknowledge that small slip-ups are normal and focus on getting back on track.

Setting Unrealistic Goals: Setting overly ambitious or unattainable goals can lead to frustration and disappointment. Set realistic, achievable goals and celebrate each milestone you reach.

Relying on Supplements or Quick Fixes: Avoid relying solely on supplements or quick-fix diets for weight loss. Focus on sustainable lifestyle changes for long-term success.

By being mindful of these common pitfalls and adopting a balanced, realistic approach to weight loss, you can enhance your chances of achieving lasting results. Consistency, self-awareness, and a positive mindset will help you overcome challenges and stay on track to reach your weight loss goals. Remember that small, sustainable changes over time can lead to significant improvements in your health and well-being.

Chapter 9: UNDERSTANDING BODY IMAGE AND SELF-ESTEEM

Body image and self-esteem play a significant role in how we perceive ourselves and approach weight loss. This chapter delves into developing a positive body image and self-acceptance, understanding the impact of self-esteem on weight loss success, and cultivating a healthy relationship with yourself.

Developing A Positive Body Image And Self-Acceptance

Developing a positive body image and self-acceptance is a transformative process that can greatly impact your overall well-being and confidence. Embracing your body and accepting yourself for who you are are essential steps in building a healthy relationship with yourself. Here are some strategies to help you cultivate a positive body image and foster self-acceptance:

Practice Self-Compassion: Be kind and understanding to yourself, especially when dealing with negative thoughts or self-criticism. Treat yourself with the same compassion and support you would offer to a friend facing similar challenges.

Focus on What Your Body Can Do: Shift your focus from solely appearance to the capabilities and strengths of your body. Appreciate the amazing things your body allows you to do, such as moving, experiencing the world, and engaging in activities you love.

Challenge Unrealistic Standards: Recognize that societal beauty standards are often unrealistic and unattainable for most people. Focus on being the best version of yourself rather than striving for an idealized image.

Surround Yourself with Positive Influences: Seek out positive influences, such as body-positive role models, uplifting social media accounts, or supportive friends and family members who celebrate your uniqueness.

Avoid Body Comparison: Avoid comparing your body to others, as it can lead to feelings of inadequacy and self-doubt. Remember that everyone's body is different, and comparison hinders self-acceptance.

Practice Mindful Self-Reflection: Take time to reflect on your thoughts and emotions related to body image. Identify negative thought patterns and replace them with positive affirmations.

Acknowledge Your Progress: Celebrate your progress and accomplishments, no matter how small they may seem. Acknowledging achievements boosts self-esteem and fosters a positive body image.

Engage in Positive Self-Talk: Replace self-critical thoughts with positive self-talk. Encourage yourself and remind yourself of your worth beyond physical appearance.

Wear Clothes That Make You Feel Good: Choose clothes that make you feel comfortable and confident. Dressing in a way that aligns with your style and body shape can enhance body positivity.

Engage in Activities You Love: Participate in activities and hobbies that bring joy and fulfillment. Engaging in enjoyable pursuits shifts the focus from appearance to personal happiness.

Recognize Media Influence: Be mindful of media content that promotes unrealistic beauty standards. Limit exposure to such content and instead consume media that promotes body diversity and inclusivity.

Seek Professional Support: If negative body image significantly impacts your mental well-being, consider seeking support from a therapist or counselor who specializes in body image issues.

Remember that developing a positive body image and self-acceptance is a journey, and it's normal to have ups and downs. Be patient with yourself, and recognize that self-acceptance is a continuous process. Embrace your uniqueness, celebrate your body, and cultivate a loving relationship with yourself to experience greater self-confidence and improved overall well-being.

The Impact Of Self-Esteem On Weight Loss Success

Self-esteem plays a crucial role in weight loss success, as it influences your attitude, motivation, and commitment to making positive lifestyle changes. How you perceive yourself and your abilities can significantly impact your weight loss journey in the following ways:

Motivation and Resilience: High self-esteem can lead to greater motivation and resilience when facing challenges during the weight loss process. Believing in your abilities to overcome obstacles can keep you on track even when progress is slow.

Confidence in Making Healthy Choices: Positive self-esteem empowers you to make confident and informed choices for your well-being. When you believe in your worth, you're more likely to prioritize self-care, make healthier food choices, and engage in regular exercise.

Goal Setting and Achievement: People with higher self-esteem tend to set more realistic and achievable weight loss goals. They are also more likely to celebrate their achievements along the way, reinforcing positive behaviors.

Accepting Imperfections: A positive self-image allows you to embrace imperfections and setbacks as part of the weight loss journey. Rather than feeling defeated, you can view setbacks as learning opportunities and continue to progress.

Avoiding Emotional Eating: Individuals with higher self-esteem are less likely to turn to food for comfort during times of stress or emotional distress. They have healthier coping mechanisms and are better equipped to manage emotions without resorting to emotional eating.

Body Image and Self-Care: Positive self-esteem is associated with a healthier body image. When you feel good about yourself, you are more likely to engage in self-care activities, nurturing your body and mind.

Self-Efficacy: Self-esteem influences self-efficacy, which is the belief in your ability to accomplish specific tasks or goals. Higher self-efficacy translates to greater confidence in your capacity to achieve weight loss success.

Perseverance: People with higher self-esteem are more likely to persevere through difficult times and continue making positive changes, even when the going gets tough.

Reducing Self-Sabotaging Behaviors: Lower self-esteem can lead to self-sabotaging behaviors, such as negative self-talk, self-doubt, and giving up on goals. Conversely, higher self-esteem reduces these behaviors, promoting healthier choices.

Maintenance of Weight Loss: After achieving weight loss goals, self-esteem plays a role in maintaining the results. Individuals with positive self-esteem are more likely to sustain healthy habits and avoid weight regain.

It's important to note that self-esteem is not fixed and can be cultivated and improved over time. Building a positive self-image and belief in your abilities are essential aspects of the weight loss journey. If you struggle with self-esteem issues that impact your weight loss progress, consider seeking support from a therapist or counselor. A professional can provide guidance and help you develop a healthier relationship with yourself, ultimately supporting your weight loss success and overall well-being.

Cultivating A Healthy Relationship With Yourself

Cultivating a healthy relationship with yourself is a transformative and empowering journey that can positively impact every aspect of your life, including your weight loss journey. A healthy relationship with yourself involves self-acceptance, self-compassion, and a deep understanding of your worth. Here are some steps to help you cultivate a healthy relationship with yourself:

Practice Self-Awareness: Take time to explore your thoughts, feelings, and behaviors. Be honest with yourself and acknowledge areas that need improvement or self-compassion.

Embrace Self-Acceptance: Accept yourself as you are, with all your strengths and imperfections. Recognize that nobody is perfect, and it's okay to have flaws.

Challenge Self-Criticism: When you catch yourself engaging in self-critical thoughts, challenge them with positive affirmations and compassionate self-talk.

Set Boundaries: Learn to set healthy boundaries in your relationships, both with yourself and others. Saying no when necessary and prioritizing your needs is essential for self-care.

Engage in Self-Care: Prioritize self-care activities that nourish your body, mind, and soul. This can include practicing mindfulness, engaging in hobbies, spending time in nature, or enjoying a relaxing bath.

Practice Self-Compassion: Be kind and understanding to yourself, especially during challenging times. Treat yourself with the same kindness and compassion you would offer to a friend.

Celebrate Your Accomplishments: Recognize and celebrate your achievements, no matter how small. Celebrating progress reinforces positive behaviors and boosts self-esteem.

Forgive Yourself: Understand that making mistakes is a natural part of being human. Forgive yourself for past shortcomings and use them as opportunities for growth and learning.

Cultivate Positive Relationships: Surround yourself with supportive and uplifting people who appreciate and celebrate you for who you are.

Focus on Positive Qualities: Acknowledge your positive qualities and strengths. Building a positive self-image enhances self-esteem and overall well-being.

Let Go of Comparison: Avoid comparing yourself to others. Focus on your own progress and journey, recognizing that everyone has their unique path.

Set Realistic Goals: Set achievable and realistic goals for yourself. Celebrate your progress and avoid self-criticism for not reaching perfection.

Engage in Activities You Love: Participate in activities and hobbies that bring you joy and fulfillment. Engaging in activities you love fosters a deeper connection with yourself.

Practice Gratitude: Cultivate gratitude for what you have in your life. Gratitude shifts your focus from what's lacking to what's abundant.

Remember that cultivating a healthy relationship with yourself is an ongoing process, and it's okay to have ups and downs. Be patient and gentle with yourself, and celebrate the progress you make in building a positive and loving relationship with the most important person in your life – yourself. As you nurture this connection, you'll find greater self-confidence, resilience, and happiness, which will positively influence your weight loss journey and all areas of your life.

CHAPTER 10: MINDFULNESS AND MENTAL HEALTH

Mindfulness and mental health play a critical role in achieving sustainable weight loss and overall well-being. This chapter explores the benefits of embracing mindfulness practices for weight loss and health, coping with emotional challenges and stress, and understanding the profound connection between mental health and physical well-being.

Embracing Mindfulness Practices For Weight Loss And Health

Embracing mindfulness practices for weight loss and health can be a transformative approach to achieving sustainable results and overall well-being. Mindfulness involves being fully present, non-judgmentally aware of your thoughts, feelings, and sensations. By incorporating mindfulness into your weight loss journey, you can develop a deeper connection with your body, emotions, and behaviors. Here are some ways to embrace mindfulness practices for weight loss and health:

Mindful Eating: Pay attention to the taste, smell, and texture of your food. Slow down during meals, chew mindfully, and savor each bite. This practice can help you recognize hunger cues and feelings of fullness, preventing overeating.

Keep a Food Journal: Maintain a food journal to track not only what you eat but also your emotions and circumstances surrounding eating. This can help you identify patterns of emotional eating and mindless snacking.

Practice Mindful Movement: Engage in physical activities like yoga, tai chi, or walking meditation. These practices promote mind-body connection, reduce stress, and improve overall well-being.

Breathing Exercises: Incorporate deep breathing exercises into your daily routine. Focus on your breath, and this can help calm your nervous system, reduce stress, and enhance self-awareness.

Practice Mindful Self-Compassion: Be kind and understanding to yourself during your weight loss journey. Treat yourself with the same compassion you would offer to a friend facing similar challenges.

Embrace Mindful Cooking: Pay attention to the ingredients and cooking process. Engaging in mindful cooking can deepen your connection with food and foster a healthier relationship with eating.

Engage Your Senses: Use all your senses during mealtime. Notice the colors, smells, and flavors of your food, making the experience more enjoyable and satisfying.

Mindful Snacking: Be mindful of your snacking habits. Ask yourself if you are truly hungry or eating out of boredom or stress.

Stay Present during Exercise: During workouts, focus on the sensations in your body, breathing, and movement. Mindful exercise can improve your connection with your body and make workouts more enjoyable.

Practice Gratitude: Cultivate gratitude for the nourishing food you consume and the efforts you put into your health. Gratitude practices enhance positive emotions and promote a healthier mindset.

By embracing mindfulness practices for weight loss and health, you become more attuned to your body's needs, emotions, and triggers. This heightened self-awareness can lead to making healthier choices, developing a more positive relationship with food, and reducing emotional eating. Mindfulness practices also help reduce stress, enhance overall well-being, and support your weight loss journey in a sustainable and compassionate way. Remember that mindfulness is a skill that requires practice, patience, and consistency, and over time, it can profoundly impact your physical and mental health, leading to positive and lasting changes.

Coping With Emotional Challenges And Stress

Coping with emotional challenges and stress is crucial for maintaining well-being and supporting your weight loss journey. Emotional challenges, such as stress, anxiety, boredom, or sadness, can often trigger emotional eating or unhealthy behaviors, hindering your progress. Here are some effective strategies to help you cope with emotional challenges and manage stress:

Mindfulness and Deep Breathing: Practice mindfulness and deep breathing exercises to bring your awareness to the present moment. Deep breathing can activate your body's relaxation response, reducing stress and promoting emotional balance.

Identify Triggers: Be aware of situations or emotions that trigger emotional eating or stress. Identifying your triggers can help you find healthier ways to cope with these challenges.

Practice Emotional Awareness: Develop emotional awareness by recognizing and labeling your feelings. Accept that it's normal to experience emotions and give yourself permission to feel them without judgment.

Reach Out for Support: Talk to a friend, family member, or counselor about your emotions and stress. Sharing your feelings with someone you trust can provide relief and support.

Engage in Physical Activity: Exercise is a powerful stress-reliever and mood-booster. Engage in activities you enjoy, such as walking, dancing, or yoga, to release tension and improve your mood.

Practice Self-Compassion: Be kind to yourself during challenging times. Avoid self-criticism and practice self-compassion, understanding that everyone faces emotional challenges and setbacks.

Distract Yourself: Find healthy distractions when you feel overwhelmed by emotions. Engage in hobbies, listen to music, read a book, or take a walk to shift your focus.

Seek Professional Help: If emotional challenges or stress are impacting your daily life and well-being, consider seeking support from a mental health professional. Therapy can provide valuable tools to cope with stress and emotions effectively.

Practice Gratitude: Cultivate gratitude for the positive aspects of your life. Keeping a gratitude journal can shift your focus from stress to what you appreciate, improving your overall outlook.

Set Realistic Expectations: Avoid placing too much pressure on yourself. Set realistic expectations for your weight loss journey and recognize that progress takes time.

Time Management: Organize your daily tasks and responsibilities to reduce stress. Prioritize self-care and allocate time for relaxation and activities that bring you joy.

Limit Exposure to Stressors: If possible, limit exposure to stressful situations or people that contribute to emotional challenges. Create boundaries to protect your emotional well-being.

Remember that emotional challenges and stress are a normal part of life. Coping effectively with them allows you to navigate your weight loss journey more successfully. By developing healthy coping mechanisms, seeking support when needed, and practicing self-compassion, you can better manage emotional challenges and create a positive and balanced approach to weight loss and overall well-being.

The Connection Between Mental Health And Physical Well-being

The connection between mental health and physical well-being is profound and complex. The state of our mental health can significantly impact our physical health, and vice versa. Here are some ways in which mental health and physical well-being are interconnected:

Stress and Hormonal Response: Mental health issues like chronic stress, anxiety, and depression can trigger the release of stress hormones such as cortisol and adrenaline. Prolonged exposure to these hormones can lead to various physical health problems, including high blood pressure, weakened immune function, and an increased risk of chronic diseases.

Immune System Function: Mental health can influence the strength of our immune system. Chronic stress and negative emotions can weaken the immune response, making us more susceptible to infections and illnesses.

Sleep Quality: Mental health issues can negatively impact sleep quality and quantity. Poor sleep, in turn, affects our physical health, increasing the risk of obesity, cardiovascular diseases, and other health conditions.

Emotional Eating: Emotional challenges, such as stress, anxiety, or sadness, can trigger emotional eating as a coping mechanism. This behavior can lead to weight gain and hinder weight loss efforts.

Substance Use: Mental health disorders can increase the risk of substance abuse. Substance abuse, in turn, can harm physical health and lead to various health complications.

Inflammation: Chronic stress and negative emotions can contribute to increased inflammation in the body. Chronic inflammation is associated with several health issues, including cardiovascular diseases, diabetes, and autoimmune disorders.

Cognitive Function: Mental health plays a crucial role in cognitive function and memory. Cognitive decline due to mental health issues can impact physical health, affecting daily activities and quality of life.

Pain Perception: Mental health can influence how we perceive and manage pain. Individuals with mental health challenges may experience heightened pain sensitivity or find it more challenging to cope with chronic pain.

Physical Activity: Engaging in regular physical activity is beneficial for mental health, as it can reduce stress, improve mood, and enhance cognitive function. Conversely, physical activity also promotes physical well-being and overall health.

Resilience and Coping: Good mental health improves resilience, enabling individuals to cope with life's challenges and make healthier choices for their physical well-being.

Medication Adherence: Mental health disorders can impact medication adherence, leading to suboptimal management of physical health conditions.

Social Interaction: Mental health influences social interactions and relationships, which play a crucial role in overall well-being. Social support is essential for maintaining physical health and emotional well-being.

It's essential to recognize the interconnectedness of mental health and physical well-being and prioritize both aspects of health. Taking care of our mental health through stress management, seeking support when needed, and practicing self-care can positively impact our physical health and contribute to a more balanced and fulfilling life. Similarly, maintaining good physical health through regular exercise, nutritious diet, and adequate sleep can promote positive mental well-being and emotional resilience. By addressing mental and physical health holistically, we can work towards achieving overall well-being and a higher quality of life.

CHAPTER 11: NAVIGATING SOCIAL SITUATIONS AND CHALLENGES

Social events and gatherings can present unique challenges when it comes to staying on track with your weight loss goals. This chapter provides strategies for navigating such situations, overcoming temptations, and effectively communicating your weight loss journey with others.

Strategies For Staying On Track During Social Events And Gatherings

Staying on track during social events and gatherings is essential for maintaining your weight loss progress and overall health goals. These occasions often present tempting food options and may disrupt your regular routine. However, with some strategic planning and mindful choices, you can navigate these situations successfully. Here are some effective strategies to help you stay on track:

Plan Ahead: Before attending a social event, find out if there will be a meal or snacks served. Knowing the menu in advance can help you plan your food choices and avoid impulsive decisions.

Eat a Balanced Meal Beforehand: Consider having a balanced and nutritious meal before the event to avoid arriving hungry. This can help you make healthier choices and prevent overeating.

Bring a Healthy Dish: Offer to bring a dish to share with others that aligns with your dietary preferences. Bringing a nutritious option ensures you have a healthy choice available.

Practice Mindful Eating: Be mindful of your food choices and portion sizes during the event. Savor each bite, eat slowly, and pay attention to hunger and fullness cues.

Focus on Social Connections: Concentrate on connecting with others rather than solely on food. Engaging in meaningful conversations can reduce the emphasis on eating.

Choose Wisely from the Menu: If there's a menu, opt for healthier options like salads, lean proteins, and vegetables. Choose grilled, baked, or steamed dishes instead of fried or heavily sauced items.

Be Selective with Alcohol: Limit your alcohol consumption, as it can add empty calories and lower inhibitions, leading to less mindful eating.

Stay Hydrated: Drink water throughout the event to stay hydrated and help control your appetite.

Set Boundaries: Politely decline offers of food or drinks that don't align with your goals. Practice setting boundaries to protect your commitment to your health.

Practice Portion Control: If there are indulgent treats you'd like to try, practice portion control. Savor a small portion and then focus on other healthier options.

Avoid Grazing: Refrain from continuously grazing on snacks or appetizers. Instead, create a balanced plate of food and enjoy it mindfully.

Bring Healthy Snacks: If you know there might be limited healthy options available, consider bringing your own nutritious snacks to the event.

Seek Support: If possible, attend social events with friends or family who support your health goals. Surrounding yourself with supportive individuals can help you stay on track.

Plan for Desserts: If you anticipate desserts being served, plan ahead for a small indulgence or consider healthier dessert alternatives like fresh fruit.

Focus on Non-Food Activities: Engage in non-food-related activities during the event, such as dancing, playing games, or taking a walk.

By implementing these strategies, you can enjoy social events and gatherings while staying committed to your weight loss and health goals. Remember that mindful choices and planning ahead can make a significant difference in maintaining your progress and ensuring a positive and enjoyable experience at social occasions.

Overcoming Temptations And Staying Committed To Your Goals

Overcoming temptations and staying committed to your goals is a crucial aspect of achieving long-term success in your weight loss journey. Temptations can arise in various forms, such as unhealthy food choices, lack of motivation, or encountering setbacks. Here are some effective strategies to help you overcome temptations and maintain your commitment to your goals:

Identify Triggers: Recognize the specific situations, emotions, or events that trigger temptations. Understanding your triggers allows you to develop targeted strategies to cope with them.

Visualize Success: Envision yourself achieving your weight loss goals and experiencing the benefits of a healthier lifestyle. This positive visualization can reinforce your commitment and motivate you to stay on track.

Find Healthy Alternatives: Seek out healthier alternatives for your favorite treats or comfort foods. Experiment with nutritious and satisfying alternatives to curb cravings.

Practice Self-Control: When faced with temptations, take a moment to pause and reflect on your goals. Remind yourself of the reasons you started your weight loss journey and the positive changes you've experienced.

Set Realistic Goals: Set achievable and realistic goals to avoid feeling overwhelmed or discouraged. Celebrate each milestone, no matter how small, as it reinforces your commitment.

Learn from Slip-Ups: If you give in to temptations, view it as a learning experience rather than a failure. Identify what triggered the slip-up and develop strategies to prevent it from happening again.

Create a Support System: Surround yourself with supportive friends, family, or a weight loss group who can provide encouragement and understanding during challenging times.

Accountability Partners: Share your goals with a trusted friend or family member who can help hold you accountable and provide motivation when needed.

Focus on Non-Food Rewards: Find non-food rewards to celebrate your achievements. Treat yourself to a massage, a new workout outfit, or a hobby you enjoy.

Practice Mindfulness: Be mindful of your thoughts and emotions around temptations. Recognize cravings as temporary sensations that will pass with time.

Stay Away from Triggers: If certain foods or environments consistently trigger temptations, try to avoid them when possible.

Embrace the Process: Understand that setbacks and temptations are a natural part of any journey. Embrace the process of growth and view challenges as opportunities for improvement.

Keep a Journal: Maintain a journal to track your progress, thoughts, and emotions. Reflecting on your journey can provide valuable insights and motivation.

Stay Positive and Patient: Be kind to yourself and practice self-compassion. Stay positive and patient with your progress, understanding that sustainable change takes time.

Seek Professional Support: If you find it challenging to overcome temptations on your own, consider seeking guidance from a health professional or a therapist who specializes in weight loss and behavior change.

Remember that staying committed to your goals is a continuous effort that involves both mental and physical aspects. By implementing these strategies and building a resilient mindset, you can navigate temptations and stay focused on your weight loss journey, leading to lasting and positive changes in your life.

Communicating Your Weight Loss Journey With Others

Communicating your weight loss journey with others can be a rewarding and empowering experience. Sharing your progress, challenges, and goals can create a support system that encourages and motivates you throughout your weight loss journey. However, it's essential to approach these conversations thoughtfully and assertively to ensure a positive and supportive response from those around you. Here are some tips for effectively communicating your weight loss journey with others:

Be Confident and Proud: Embrace your weight loss journey with confidence and pride. Share your progress and achievements with enthusiasm, demonstrating your commitment to your goals.

Choose the Right Time and Place: Select an appropriate time and place to discuss your weight loss journey with others. Avoid sensitive situations or gatherings where food is the primary focus.

Share Your Motivation: Explain the reasons behind your decision to embark on this journey. Whether it's improving your health, increasing energy levels, or boosting self-esteem, sharing your motivations can help others understand your commitment.

Be Honest and Transparent: Be open and honest about your progress, both the successes and challenges you've encountered. Honesty creates a sense of authenticity and vulnerability that can deepen connections with others.

Set Boundaries: If certain topics or comments make you uncomfortable, kindly set boundaries with others to ensure they respect your journey.

Educate Others: Educate those close to you about the importance of your health goals and how they can support you. Help them understand your dietary choices and exercise routines.

Seek Support: Share your weight loss goals with supportive friends or family members who can provide encouragement and understanding.

Address Potential Misunderstandings: Some people might have misconceptions or misguided opinions about weight loss. Be prepared to address and correct any misunderstandings they may have.

Be Patient with Responses: Understand that not everyone will share your enthusiasm or understand your journey right away. Be patient with others' responses and allow them time to adjust to your changes.

Focus on Health, Not Appearance: Emphasize that your weight loss journey is primarily about improving your health and well-being rather than solely focused on appearance.

Encourage Positive Support: Communicate your need for positive support and encouragement. Request that others avoid negative comments or judgments that may hinder your progress.

Lead by Example: Show others the positive changes you're experiencing through your commitment to your goals. Leading by example can inspire and motivate others to adopt healthier habits too.

Express Gratitude: Thank those who have been supportive of your journey. Expressing gratitude reinforces their positive impact on your life.

Remember that not everyone will fully understand or support your weight loss journey, and that's okay. Focus on the individuals who are encouraging and uplifting, and surround yourself with a positive and understanding support system. Communicating your weight loss journey with others can deepen connections, provide motivation, and make your path to a healthier lifestyle more enjoyable and fulfilling.

CHAPTER 12: CELEBRATING YOUR SUCCESS AND MAINTAINING MOTIVATION

After making progress in your weight loss journey, it's essential to recognize and celebrate your achievements. This chapter focuses on acknowledging milestones, setting new goals, and finding fulfillment and joy in your healthier lifestyle to maintain your motivation for long-term success.

Recognizing And Celebrating Milestones In Your Journey

Take the time to acknowledge and celebrate your accomplishments along the way. Whether it's reaching a specific weight loss milestone, consistently sticking to your exercise routine, or adopting healthier eating habits, each achievement deserves recognition. Celebrating milestones can:

Boost Your Confidence: Recognizing your progress reinforces your belief in your capabilities and strengthens your determination to keep going.

Provide Positive Reinforcement: Celebrating your achievements positively reinforces the healthy behaviors you've cultivated, making them more likely to become lasting habits.

Motivate You to Continue: Celebrating milestones inspires you to continue your journey and work towards even more significant achievements.

Setting New Goals And Continuing To Improve

As you reach milestones, it's crucial to set new goals to maintain your motivation and sense of purpose. Setting new goals:

Keeps You Engaged: Having new objectives to work towards keeps your journey exciting and prevents complacency.

Creates a Sense of Direction: Clear goals provide a roadmap for your continued progress and improvement.

Allows for Continuous Growth: Setting new challenges enables you to grow and improve physically and mentally.

Finding Fulfillment And Joy In Your Healthier Lifestyle

Embrace the positive changes you've made in your life and find fulfillment in your healthier lifestyle:

Discover New Activities: Explore physical activities or hobbies that bring you joy and align with your goals.

Nourish Your Body and Mind: Prioritize self-care and nourishment to maintain your overall well-being.

Practice Gratitude: Cultivate gratitude for the progress you've made and the positive impact on your life.

Surround Yourself with Support: Stay connected with friends and family who support your journey and inspire you to keep going.

Reflect on Your Journey: Reflect on how far you've come and the positive changes you've experienced. Remembering your transformation can fuel your motivation.

Focus on Non-Scale Victories: Celebrate non-scale victories like increased energy, improved mood, or better sleep, as they are equally important indicators of success.

Be Patient and Compassionate: Understand that progress may not always be linear. Be patient with yourself and practice self-compassion during challenging times.

Share Your Journey: Share your success with others, as your story can inspire and motivate those on a similar path.

By recognizing milestones, setting new goals, and finding fulfillment in your healthier lifestyle, you can maintain your motivation and enthusiasm for your weight loss journey. Celebrating your success along the way will help you stay committed and inspired to continue making positive changes for a happier and healthier life. Remember that the journey is ongoing, and with each milestone, you pave the way for a more empowered and fulfilling future.

CONCLUSION

As we come to the end of "Lose Weight, Gain Health: Your Journey to a Better You," I hope this book has been a source of inspiration, guidance, and empowerment on your path to a healthier and happier life. Throughout this journey, you have learned that weight loss is not merely about shedding pounds; it's about gaining a profound understanding of yourself, nurturing a positive relationship with your body, and embracing a sustainable and mindful approach to health and well-being.

Remember that your transformation is a journey, not a destination. It's about progress, not perfection. Each step you've taken, every milestone you've reached, and every challenge you've overcome has contributed to your growth and success. Embrace the power of self-compassion, as it will sustain you during moments of difficulty and remind you that you are worthy of love and care, regardless of the number on the scale.

As you move forward, continue to practice mindful eating, savoring each bite and listening to your body's signals of hunger and fullness. Cherish the moments of physical activity, finding joy in movement, and discovering new ways to keep your body active and strong.

Maintain your focus on nurturing your mental and emotional well-being, as a healthy mind is the foundation for a healthy body. Take time for self-reflection, practice gratitude, and surround yourself with supportive individuals who uplift and encourage you on your journey.

It's essential to celebrate every victory, no matter how small, and remember that setbacks are opportunities for growth and learning. Embrace the journey, knowing that the road may have twists and turns, but each step you take brings you closer to becoming the best version of yourself.

As you continue on this transformative path, always remember that you are deserving of good health, happiness, and fulfillment. You have the strength and resilience within you to overcome any challenge and achieve your goals. Keep the flame of motivation alive, and never forget that you possess the power to create positive and lasting change in your life.

I am deeply grateful for joining you on this transformative journey. Remember, you are not alone; you have the support of this book and the knowledge gained from it. Embrace your uniqueness, cherish your progress, and trust in yourself as you move forward, gaining health and becoming a better you.

May your life be filled with abundant health, joy, and fulfillment. Your journey to lose weight, gain health, and become the best version of yourself continues, and I am excited to witness the remarkable impact you will create in your life and the lives of those around you.

Cheers to your vibrant, healthy, and extraordinary future!
The journey has just begun.